THE TYPE 2 DIABETES REVERSAL CODE

Simple Natural Ways to Prevent and Reverse It

by

Dr. Henry M. Daniel

Table of content

Disclaimer

As a consequence of the information or material in this book, the author expressly disclaims responsibility for any loss or harm incurred by any individual. Only instructional goals should be served by the content in this book. The medical and health information in this book is offered solely for general educational and informative reasons and does not replace the advice of a healthcare provider.

Therefore, we urge you to speak with the right experts before acting in any way based on this material.

Introduction

Through strong lifestyle modifications, such as dietary adjustments, dietary supplements, exercise, and stress reduction - diabetes and insulin resistance can be avoided and frequently reversed.

High blood sugar is a symptom of the chronic metabolic illness diabetes. When you have diabetes, your body either produces insufficient hormones or is unable to use the hormones it does produce properly.

The most common type of diabetes, type 2, arises when the body is unable to generate enough insulin or develops a resistance to it, making it challenging for the body to efficiently absorb insulin from the blood.

Although there is no known cure for type 2 diabetes, some people may be able to reverse it, according to studies. By changing your diet and decreasing weight, you might be able to attain and maintain normal blood sugar levels without using medication.

This doesn't always mean you've recovered completely. Diabetes type 2 is a chronic condition. Even if you are in remission, which means you are not taking any medication and your blood sugar levels remain within a safe range, there is still a chance that symptoms might return. However, some people with diabetes can go for years without having problems controlling their blood sugar levels or suffering the related health concerns.

How therefore may diabetes be cured?

Losing weight seemed to be the key. Exercise, stress management, dietary changes, and weight loss can sometimes help you manage your diabetes and even help you live a diabetes-free life, especially if you've only had the disease for a short while and haven't required insulin.

If you have type 2 diabetes, cells that help your body regulate your blood sugar cease working correctly. Contrary to what physicians formerly thought, researchers have discovered that certain cells may regenerate. People who lost weight had lower liver and pancreatic fat levels, which in some cases allowed the pancreatic beta cells to reactivate and begin producing insulin and regulating blood sugar.

Type 2 Diabetes

Type 2 diabetes is a disorder that develops when the body's ability to control and utilize sugar as fuel is compromised. Glucose is another name for same sugar. Too much sugar is constantly moving through the blood as a result of this chronic illness. Eventually, problems with the brain, immunological, and cardiovascular systems can result from excessive blood sugar levels.

Generally speaking, type 2 diabetes has two issues. Insulin, a hormone that controls how quickly sugar enters cells, is not produced by the pancreas in sufficient amounts. Additionally, cells absorb less sugar and have a weak insulin response.

What Causes Type 2 Diabetes?

The most prevalent form of diabetes, type 2, is brought on by issues with the insulin hormone. It is frequently associated with being obese or inactive, having a family history of type 2 diabetes, and a number of lifestyle variables, such as obesity and inactivity. The most frequent cause of type 2 diabetes is insulin resistance. High blood sugar levels, exhaustion, and weight gain are some of the signs and symptoms of type 2 diabetes that can appear gradually over time. While some people can maintain their blood glucose levels with healthy nutrition and exercise, others might require medication or insulin to do so.

Type 2 Diabetes symptoms

Type 2 diabetes symptoms frequently appear gradually. In fact, you may have type 2 diabetes for years without realizing it. When symptoms do exist, they may consist of:

- More satiety or hunger.
- Lots of urine.
- An increase in appetite.

- Loss of weight without meaning to.

- Fatigue.

- Fuzzy vision.

- Wounds that are heal slowly.

- Lots of infections.

- Hands or feet that tingle or are numb.

- Skin spots that have darkened, usually in the armpit and neck area

Simple Steps to Reverse Diabetes Type 2

Modify Your Diet

Eating in a way that maintains a healthy blood sugar level, reduces inflammation and oxidative stress, and supports liver detoxification is essential for preventing and treating insulin resistance and diabetes.

A whole foods diet high in fiber, packed with colorful fruits and vegetables, low in sugar and wheat, and with a low glycemic load is the foundation of this eating pattern. It is a diet that consists of foods that are detoxifying, anti-inflammatory, and antioxidant. There is also a lot of omega-3 fats, olive oil, soy products, beans, nuts, and seeds.

All of these foods help prevent and treat diabetes and insulin resistance. This food regimen maintains a healthy metabolism, activates all required gene signals, and protects against aging and age-related disorders.

Exercise

The enhancement of insulin sensitivity depends on exercise. It helps to reduce central body fat while improving sugar metabolism. Regular exercise can help you avoid complications from diabetes, manage it, and even reverse it.

You ought to aim to walk for 30 minutes every day. Walking after dinner can help reduce blood sugar levels.

Interval training can also boost mitochondrial function and metabolism. You can burn more calories and energy even when you aren't exercising thanks to its assistance in improving the efficiency of calorie burning. This is covered in great detail in Ultra-Metabolism.

The entire blood sugar and energy metabolism of your body can be improved by strength training, which encourages muscle development and maintenance.

Take Nutritional Supplements

Nutritional supplements can be used to treat type 2 diabetes and insulin resistance. I recommend a range of dietary supplements, depending on how bad the problem is:

A mineral and vitamin supplement

Magnesium, calcium, and vitamin D

Inflammation is decreased, cholesterol is lowered, and insulin sensitivity is improved with fish oil (1,000 to 4,000 mg per day).

Magnesium is deficient in diabetics and has to be supplemented daily with 200–600 mg.

Chromium (500–1,000 mcg per day) is essential for optimum sugar metabolism.

Blood sugar levels can be lowered and stabilized with the help of vitamins C and E and other antioxidants.

A decent multivitamin should contain the B-complex vitamins because they are crucial. Increased vitamin B6 intake (50 to 150 mg per day) and for reducing diabetic neuropathy or nerve damage, and B12 consumption (1,000 to 3,000 mcg per day).

Control Stress

Stress significantly contributes to blood sugar abnormalities. It promotes the gain of belly fat, exacerbates inflammation, and eventually raises the risk of developing diabetes. Exercise, meditation, massage, biofeedback, hypnosis, guided imagery, hot baths, yoga, breathing exercises, progressive muscle relaxation, and so on are all excellent ways to unwind. Your life relies on it.

What weight loss is necessary to reverse type 2 diabetes?

Working with a professional and exercising extreme restraint when it comes to calorie intake are necessary for type 2 diabetes to be reversed. Most persons with type 2 diabetes who were able to reverse it lost 30 pounds or more. You might be able to reverse type 2 diabetes if you recently received a diagnosis by losing roughly 10% of your weight. Remission is less likely, though, as diabetes progresses and the body may start to lose its capacity to produce insulin. However, by decreasing 20% to 25% of their body weight, some persons with severe type 2 diabetes may be able to go into remission.

How do foods affect the synthesis of Insulin?

All carbs will, at the very least, raise your blood insulin levels. I view type 2 diabetes as a type of "carbohydrate intolerance" because of this. Although considerably less effectively, protein can also increase levels. Fat is the only macronutrient that maintains steady levels of insulin and, consequently, blood sugar. Therefore, if you want to lower your insulin levels, you should consume less of these carbohydrates and more of healthy, natural fats.

Think about nuts, seeds, avocados, extra virgin olive oil, whole eggs, and omega 3 fats (found in almonds, flaxseed, and cold-water fish like wild salmon, herring, mackerel, and tuna) when I say healthy, natural fat.

And when I talk about cutting back on some carbohydrates, I primarily mean processed carbohydrates like pasta, rice, and bread. Broccoli, cabbage, and other non-starchy veggies are ok and can be consumed in large quantities. If you're attempting to cut back on your intake of carbohydrates, try to stick to low-carb fruits like rhubarb, watermelon, berries, peaches, and blackberries.

What ought to include on a Type 2 diabetic food plan?

A Type 2 diabetes meal plan should often include lean proteins with less saturated fat including chicken, eggs, and shellfish. Tofu, almonds, and beans are a few examples of plant proteins.

Carbohydrates that have had little processing: Refined carbohydrates like white bread, pasta, and potatoes can quickly raise your blood sugar. Select carbohydrates that raise blood sugar more gradually, such as whole grains like oatmeal, brown rice, and whole-grain pasta.

Devoid of salt: Your blood pressure might rise if you consume too much sodium or salt. By staying away from processed meals like those in cans or packages, you can reduce your salt intake. Instead of using salad dressing, use spices without salt and healthy oils.

Sugars not added: Steer clear of sweet meals and beverages like soda, pies, and cakes.

The Risk Factors of Diabetes Type 2

Weight: Being overweight or obese is a serious concern.

dispersion of fat. A higher risk is indicated by storing fat mostly in the belly as opposed to the hips and thighs. Men with a waist measurement over 40 inches (101.6 centimeters) and women with a waist measurement above 35 inches (88.9 centimeters) have an increased chance of developing type 2 diabetes.

Prediabetes: When blood sugar levels are above normal but not high enough to be considered diabetic, the condition is called prediabetes. Prediabetes frequently develops into type 2 diabetes if left untreated.

Family background: If a parent or sibling has the disease, a person is more likely to get type 2 diabetes themselves.

Inactivity: The danger increases with a person's level of inactivity. Exercise aids in weight management, burns glucose as fuel, and increases insulin sensitivity in cells.

levels of blood lipids: Low levels of high-density lipoprotein (HDL) cholesterol, or the "good" cholesterol, and high levels of triglycerides are linked to an increased risk.

Age: Type 2 diabetes risk rises with age, particularly beyond the age of 35.

Complications Linked To Type 2 Diabetes

Type 2 diabetes has an effect on several vital organs, including the kidneys, blood vessels, nerves, eyes, and heart. Additionally, risk factors for diabetes may raise the chance of other severe illnesses. Controlling blood sugar and managing diabetes can reduce the likelihood of these consequences and other illnesses, such as:

Neuropathy: Neuropathy is the medical term for harm to a limb's nerves. Long-term high blood sugar levels can damage or even kill nerves. As a result, there may be tingling, numbness, burning, discomfort, or even ultimate loss of sensation, which often starts at the ends of the toes or fingers and slowly moves higher.

Kidney illness: Diabetes may cause chronic renal disease or irreversible end-stage kidney disease. That could necessitate kidney transplantation or dialysis.

Eye injury: Diabetes may damage the blood vessels in the retina, potentially resulting in blindness, and also raises the risk of significant eye conditions such cataracts and glaucoma.

Slow recovery: Cuts and blisters can develop into dangerous infections that may not heal properly if left untreated. Amputations of the toe, foot, or leg may be necessary for severe injuries.

Impairment of hearing: Patients with diabetes are more prone to have hearing problems.

Apneic sleep: Obstructive sleep apnea is a common complication of type 2 diabetes. Obesity may be the root cause of several disorders.

Dementia: Alzheimer's disease and other kinds of dementia appear to be more common among people with type 2 diabetes. Poor blood sugar control is also linked to cognitive decline, including memory loss.

Conclusion

Type 2 diabetes can enter remission with treatment. The end of diabetes is not, however, indicated by remission. To maintain remission, you must control and keep an eye on your blood sugar levels.

Type 1 and type 2 diabetes are very different from one another. The former is a result of dangerously high insulin levels, which in turn cause insulin resistance and a variety of major health problems, whereas the latter is characterized by low insulin levels. It's comforting to know that type 2 diabetes is reversible. You'll be well on your road to recovery if you combine cutting off carbs with intermittent fasting and a change in diet.

Your outlook if you have Type 2 diabetes relies on how effectively you control your blood sugar levels. Diabetes type 2 is reversible. You can control your blood sugar by engaging in regular exercise and eating a balanced diet. You could also require insulin or medicine. If you have Type 2 diabetes, you should routinely check your blood sugar at home and keep in constant contact with your doctor.